Natural Remedies for Warts

"THE NATURAL SECRETS TO REMOVE WARTS IN 5 MINUTES A DAY"

By Charles Silverman N.D.

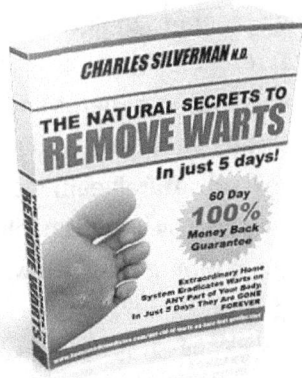

1

About:

Charles Silverman N.D., a Naturalist and Herbalist since 1979, is the author of the Home Made Medicine e-book and the www.HomeMadeMedicine.com Web site. Charles lives in Miami, FL and has dedicated a major part of his life to the preparation of natural remedies and natural products to help people with allergies and chemical intolerance. He has traveled around the world from Canada, Germany, France, and India to the mountains of Peru and Argentina (South America) researching and studying the different domestic species of herbs and plants. His articles are published on several web sites like ezinearticles.com and naturalhealthweb.com and he is regularly interviewed by various publications and newspapers like the Montgomery News of Alabama. All his knowledge has been transferred to his web site and now to this amazing book, that takes advantage of the latest technology in order to bring you the most complete guide for home healing ever made.

Disclaimer:

Information in this book is provided for informational purposes and is not meant to substitute for the advice of your physician or health care professional. You should not use this information to diagnose or treat a health problem or disease, nor to prescribe any medication. You should read all product packaging and labels carefully. If you have or suspect that you have a medical condition, promptly contact your health care provider.   Remember that some herbs if used often may produce some minor irritations or stomach upsets. If you are allergic to ragweed or any other plant, consult your physician before taking any herbal remedy.

It is very embarrassing to have warts, but more awkward is going to the pharmacy to get an over the counter product to treat them, that is why most people search for a more private way to remove warts, without a doubt home remedies to remove warts are the answer for most of us. There are many home remedies warts below.

Warts are small benign growths on the skin, caused by a variety of related, slow-acting viruses HPV (human papilloma virus). There are at least sixty known types of HPV. Warts may appear singly or in clusters. We will talk about three types of warts and the home remedies that can take care of all of them: Common warts, plantar warts, and genital warts.

Common warts can be found anywhere on the body, but are most common on the hands, fingers elbows, forearms, knees, face, and the skin around the nails. Most often, they occur on skin that is exposed to constant friction, trauma, or abrasion. They can also occur on the larynx (the voice box) and cause hoarseness. Common warts may be flat or raised, dry or moist, and have a rough and pitted surface that is either the same color as or slightly darker than the surrounding skin. They can be as small as a pinhead or as large as small bean. Highly contagious, the virus that causes common warts is acquired through breaks in the skin. Common warts can spread if they picked, trimmed, bitten or touched, Warts on the face can spread as a result of shaving. Common warts typically do not cause pain or itching. Home remedies warts are the best solution for this embarrassing problem.

Plantar warts occur on the sales of the feet and the underside of the toes. They are bumpy white growths that may resemble calluses, except that they can be tender to the touch and often bleed if the surface is trimmed. They also often have an identifiable hard center. Plantar warts do not tend to spread to other parts of the body. Keep reading or a special home remedy for plantar warts.

Genital warts soft, moist growths found in and around the vagina, anus, penis, groin, and/or scrotum. In men, they can grow in the urethra as well. They are usually pink or red in color and resemble tiny heads of cauliflower. Genital warts most often occur in clusters, but they can appear singly as well. They are transmitted through vaginal, oral, or anal intercourse, and are highly contagious. Because the warts do not usually appear until three months or more after an individual becomes infected with the HPV that causes them, the virus can be spread before the carrier is even aware that he or she has it. Although genital warts are not cancerous, they appear to cause changes in the cervix that may be a precursor of cervical cancer. An infant born to a mother with genital warts may contract the virus. If you have genital warts, you are not alone. Between the start of the "sexual revolution" in the sixties and the late eighties, reported occurrences of these warts increased tenfold. By 1990, one million cases a year were being reported in the United States alone.

Causes & Cures for Common Warts

You don't just find them on the faces of dirty old witches and you don't get them from kissing frogs or toads. Warts are caused by a virus, just like cold sores and they can pop up on anyone.

What Are They?

Warts are small bumps of hardened skin. They can show up anywhere on the body, but you'll usually find them on your hands, feet or face. Kids get them more often than adults do - but some kids never get any warts at all. Warts don't usually hurt but they can look pretty nasty.

How Do You Get them?

You can get warts by catching a certain virus - just like catching a cold or the flu. This wart virus shows up in moist places on your skin - like small cuts or scratches around your hands or feet. You can pick up the virus very easily by touching a towel or face cloth that someone with a wart has used. They can also spread if you keep scratching them - whether they're on your own body or someone else's.

A wart is a virus classified within the Human Papilloma Viruses (HPVs), which represent a group

of more than 100 types of viruses. They are called papilloma viruses because certain types cause warts, or papillomas, which are benign (non cancerous) tumors.

HPV, commonly known as the "wart virus", is a microscopic virus particle that infects the skin.

HPV is one of the most common infections in the world, infecting approximately 40% of all Americans.

In the case of HPV, the infection is actually localized directly to the infected point in the skin, as opposed to the herpes simplex virus. Unlike HPV, the herpes virus goes through the skin and into the nerve cells, traveling up the nerve cell connection to the nerve ganglia by the spinal cord, where the virus lives. With HPV, the infection is actually in the skin.

HPV is contagious and transmitted through contact by an infected piece of skin with a non- infected piece of skin. The presumption is that the non-infected area has to have a small, perhaps microscopic, break that allows a tiny amount of tissue from the infected HPV area to get into the non-infected area, allowing an infection to set up.

Therefore, if a person with a wart anywhere on that person's body were to place that area in contact with the genitalia of the other person, this could cause the wart virus to be transmitted to the genital area of the partner. This applies to warts on fingers as well as warts on the genitals of the infected partner.

Different types of HPVs cause common warts that grow on hands and feet than those that develop around the mouth and genital area. Warts appear as single bumps or in clusters, some having a cauliflower structure.

Of the more than 100 types of HPV identified, there are more than 30 types that have the ability to infect the genital tract. These genital warts can be passed from one person to another through sexual intercourse.

Genital HPV may cause warts to appear on or around the genitals and anus of both men and women. Genital warts often occur in groups and can be very tiny or can accumulate into large masses on genital tissues. Left untreated, genital warts may eventually develop a fleshy, cauliflower-like appearance.

Human Papilloma Virus (HPV) is one of the most common causes of sexually transmitted diseases (STDs) in this country. It is estimated that as many as 40 million Americans are infected with HPV in the genital tract, and the incidence of this disease appears to be increasing.

Warts are small benign growths on the skin, caused by a variety of related, slow-acting viruses HPV (human papilloma virus). There are at least sixty known types of HPV. Warts may appear singly or in clusters. We will talk about three types of warts: Common warts, plantar warts, and genital warts.

VERRUCA VULGARIS common warts can be found anywhere on the body, but are most common on the hands, fingers elbows, forearms, knees, face, and the skin around the nails. Most often, they occur on skin that is exposed to constant friction, trauma, or abrasion. They can also occur on the larynx (the voice box) and cause hoarseness. Common warts may be flat or raised, dry or moist, and have a rough and pitted surface that is either the same color as or slightly darker than the surrounding skin. They can be as small as a pinhead or as large as small bean.

Highly contagious, the virus that causes common warts is acquired through breaks in the skin. Common warts can spread if they picked, trimmed, bitten or touched, Warts on the face can spread as a result of shaving. Common warts typically do not cause pain or itching.

Plantar warts occur on the soles of the feet and the underside of the toes. They are bumpy white growths that may resemble calluses, except that they can be tender to the touch and often bleed if the surface is trimmed. They also often have an identifiable hard center. Plantar warts do not tend to spread to other parts of the body. Plantar warts are hyperkeratotic lesions on the plantar surface. They tend to develop over areas of pressure such as the heel and ball of the foot. Plantar warts are often endophytic (ie, they grow into the deeper layers of skin because of pressure).

Although they are generally self-limited, plantar warts should be treated to lessen symptomatology, decrease duration, and reduce transmission.

Plantar warts are widespread; 7-10% of the population has plantar warts.

Plantar wart symptoms:

•Plantar warts may cause pain, particularly when walking.

•They may spread to other sites but not to histologically dissimilar areas.

Usually spread to areas that are a different kind of skin. In other words, plantar warts do not spread to the genitalia.

Plantar warts should be treated to lessen symptoms, especially pain, to decrease duration of symptoms, and to reduce transmission to others. Because the incubation period for warts is from 1-20 months, it is difficult to tell exactly when the virus was introduced into the body.

Plantar warts may cause pain, particularly when walking. Plantar warts affect females slightly more often than males.

What do plantar warts look like:

- Firm, hyperkeratotic lesions with tiny pinpoint petechiae centrally

- Smooth surface with a gray-yellow color

- Usually occur over areas of pressure or bony prominence such as the heel and ball of the foot

- Usually flat because of pressure

- Several warts may fuse to form mosaic warts

•Often difficult to differentiate warts from nonviral causes such askeratoses, lichen planus, molluscum contagiosum, corns, calluses, and foreign body or stress fractures

Hyperkeratotic tissue reveals typical punctate hemorrhages, which represent thrombosed capillaries of the papilloma.

o   Pathologic findings include acanthotic epidermis withhyperkeratosis.

o   Papillomatosis

o   Parakeratosis

Genital warts soft, moist growths found in and around the vagina, anus, penis, groin, and/or scrotum. In men, they can grow in the urethra as well. They are usually pink or red in color and resemble tiny heads of cauliflower. Genital warts most often occur in clusters, but they can appear singly as well. They are transmitted through vaginal, oral, or anal intercourse, and are highly contagious.

Because the warts do not usually appear until three months or more after an individual becomes infected with the HPV that causes them, the virus can be spread before the carrier is even aware that he or she has it. Although genital warts are not cancerous, they appear to cause changes in the cervix that may be a precursor of cervical cancer. An infant born to a mother with genital warts may contract the virus. If you have genital warts, you are not alone. Between the start of the "sexual revolution" in the sixties and the late eighties, reported occurrences of these warts increased tenfold. By 1990, one million cases a year were being reported in the United States alone.

HPV Myths and Misconceptions

One reality is that some aspects of the virus are still poorly understood, even by medical researchers. There simply are no proven answers to many common questions.

At the same time, however, much new information about HPV has been learned in recent years, reversing some previous assumptions about the virus. The result is that older publications may be inaccurate, when they mention HPV at all. Likewise, health care professionals, writers, and educators who have not kept up with recent research findings may continue to spread misconceptions.

Another difficulty is that to some degree, the overall topic of genital HPV is complex and confusing to everyone, lay person and scientist alike. Trying to simplify the facts without misrepresenting them is a challenge that the staff of HPV News understands all too well.

The result is that, unfortunately, myths and misconceptions about genital HPV abound, and in some cases do considerable harm. Bad information can cause a person to suffer terrible anxiety unnecessarily, to doubt a partner's faithfulness, or even to undergo painful and expensive treatment that could have been avoided. Most dangerous of all, misinformation may lead people to neglect a very simple procedure that saves lives.

In this issue, we take on 12 of the most common myths and misconceptions we've encountered on the topic of genital HPV. By weeding out these persistent offenders, we hope to make room for accurate information to take root and grow.

1. Myth: I'm the only person I know with HPV.

It's easy to understand why so many people hold this misunderstanding about HPV. After all, public awareness of the virus is extremely low. Most people who contact ASHA's HPV Support Program never even heard of HPV until they were diagnosed.

21

Those struggling with this troubling condition or strange new diagnosis rarely discuss it with others, since it would seem unlikely that they would understand. And others--your second-best friend, your cousin, your coworker, your neighbor across the street--likewise feel constrained to keep silent about their HPV, thinking that you wouldn't understand.

The net result is that very few people ever have the chance to place genital HPV in an accurate context, as the very common virus it really is. According to an article published in 1997 in the American Journal of Medicine, about 74 percent of Americans--nearly three out of four—have been infected with genital HPV at some point in their lives.

Among those ages 15-49, only one in four Americans has not had a genital HPV infection.

It's true that most often genital HPV produces no symptoms or illness, and so a person who has been infected may never know about it. Experts estimate that at any given time, only about 1% of all sexually active Americans have visible genital warts. Far more women have abnormal Pap smears related to HPV infection, but in many cases health care providers do not explain the link between HPV and cervical infection, perpetuating the misunderstanding.

2. Myth: Only people who have casual sex get STDs.

Even with up to 12 million Americans contracting an STD each year, many people continue to believe that only "someone else"--for example, people who have multiple partners, sex outside of marriage, or a different lifestyle--are at risk.

It is true that a higher number of sexual partners over the course of a lifetime does correlate with a higher risk for STDs, including HPV. This is not because of any moral judgment concerning "casual" sex as compared with "committed" sex, but simply because the more sexual partners you have, the more likely you will have a partner who (knowingly or unknowingly) is carrying an STD.

However, STDs can be passed along as readily in a loving, long-term relationship as in a one- night stand. And HPV is the virus to prove it. At least one study of middle-class, middle-aged women, most of them married with children, found that 21% were infected with cervical HPV. In other studies, according to Nancy Kiviat, MD, a researcher at the University of Washington, about 80% of people who have had as few as four sexual partners have been infected with HPV.

3. Myth: In a monogamous relationship, an HPV diagnosis means someone has cheated.

This myth has been responsible for a great deal of anger, confusion, and heartache. It has led many people to tragically wrong conclusions because it fails to take into account one of the most mysterious aspects of genital HPV: its ability to lie latent.

The virus can remain in the body for weeks, years, or even a lifetime, giving no sign of its presence. Or a genital HPV infection may produce warts, lesions, or cervical abnormalities after a latent period of months or even years.

As mentioned above, most people who are infected with genital HPV never know it; their virus does not call attention to itself in any way. In most cases, a person is diagnosed with HPV only because some troubling symptom drove him or her to a health care professional, or some abnormality was revealed in the course of a routine exam.

But although careful examination can identify genital HPV infection, and laboratory tests may even narrow down the identification to a specific type among the two dozen or so that inhabit the genital tract, there is simply no way to find out how long a particular infection has been in place, or to trace it back to a particular partner.

In a monogamous relationship, therefore, just as in an affair or even in an interval of no sexual relationships at all, an HPV diagnosis means only that the person contracted an HPV infection at some point in his or her life.

4. Myth: Genital warts lead to cervical cancer.

No one knows how many sleepless nights can be laid at the door of this myth. The truth, however, is that the fleshy growths we call genital warts are almost always benign. In the vast majority of cases, they do not lead to cancer, turn into cancer, or predispose a person toward developing cancer.

According to Katherine Stone, MD, a member of ASHA's HPV Scientific Advisory Committee, genital warts need not "raise a red flag with regard to cancer in anyone's mind."

There are more than 70 types of human papillomavirus, and most are quite specific in the sites they can invade and the pathology they can cause. Those most strongly associated with cancer are HPV types 16, 18, 31, 45, and, to a lesser degree, half a dozen others. These are known as the "high-risk" types, not because they usually or frequently cause cancer--in fact, cervical cancer is a rare disease in the United States today, and penile cancer even more so—but because, in the infrequent event that cancer does develop, it can usually be traced back to one of these types. Even so, it bears repeating: most women with high-risk HPV on their cervix will not develop cervical cancer.

As for ordinary genital warts, says Doug Lowy, MD, chief of the Laboratory of Cellular Oncology at the National Cancer Institute, "These are caused by HPV types that are virtually never found in cancer." These are the "low-risk" types, 6, 11, 42, 43, and 44. When not causing genital warts they may cause a transient abnormality in Pap smear results, or most often produce no symptoms at all.

In practical terms, a man with genital warts is no more likely than any other sexually active man to transmit cancer-causing HPV types to a partner. Experts do recommend that a woman exposed to genital warts--or any other STD--have regular Pap smears. This is because she may have been exposed to high-risk HPV types during unprotected sexual activity. Regular Pap tests are also recommended for any sexually active woman, since HPV infection is very common. It is worth keeping in mind that both men and women may be infected with, and infectious for, high-risk HPV, regardless of whether or not they have genital warts.

5. Myth: An abnormal Pap smear means a woman is at high risk for cervical cancer.

First of all, an abnormal Pap smear can be caused by factors other than the presence of a high-risk HPV type. When a Pap test comes back as "abnormal," it means just that: Under the microscope, the appearance of a few cells in this sample differs in some way from the classic appearance of healthy, intact cervical cells.

The difference could be due to local irritation, a non-HPV infection, a low-risk HPV type, or even a mistake in the preparation of the cell sample. To help sort out the various possibilities, a woman with an abnormal Pap smear is often asked to come back to the doctor's office and have the test repeated. Most no significant reasons for an abnormal result last only a short time, and so repeating the Pap test after a few months usually weeds these out.

Even if the result is again abnormal, this rarely means that cancer is imminent. In an overwhelming majority of cases, a truly abnormal Pap smear is due to pre-invasive disease, not invasive disease per se. Follow-up tests such as colposcopy and biopsy can help evaluate the abnormality and remove any potentially malignant cells. If further treatment is recommended, the patient and her physician usually have several options to consider, and time in which to consider them.

What if a woman with a persistently abnormal Pap smear does not receive treatment? This scenario is very unlikely in the developed countries, where the follow-up measures described above are standard practice. But even supposing that a woman went untreated after repeated abnormal Pap results, she still would have the odds on her side, because only one out of four cases of cervical lesions will progress to cancer if left on its own. And treatment is almost always successful in preventing cervical cancer if the abnormal cells are found in time.

But this very effective system of protection can work only when each woman takes responsibility for the first step herself, by having a Pap test at regular intervals. According to the National Cancer Institute, about half of women with newly diagnosed cervical cancer have never had a Pap smear, and another 10% have not had a smear in the past five years.

6. Myth: If I have genital warts or dysplasia, I will have recurrences for the rest of my life.

Warts and dysplasia do recur in some cases, but by no means all. When they recur, they show varying persistence: Some people experience just one more episode and others several. The good news for most people is that with time, the immune system seems to gain some mastery over the virus, making recurrences less frequent and often eliminating them entirely within about two years.

The limiting factor here is the state of the immune system itself. According to Thomas Sedlacek, MD, a member of ASHA's Scientific Advisory Committee and adjunct professor of obstetrics and gynecology at Allegheny University, if an individual's immune system is impaired--by the use of certain medications, by HIV infection, or by some temporary trauma such as excessive stress, serious illness, or surgery--it may be unable to prevent a recurrence. However, if the immune system is weakened only temporarily, most likely the recurrence will be short-lived.

The concern about life-long recurrences may be based on a misconception rather than a myth.

It's true that at present there is no known cure for genital human papillomavirus. As a virus, it will remain in the infected person's cells for an indefinite time--most often in a latent state but occasionally producing symptoms or disease, as we have discussed elsewhere.

Recent studies from the Albert Einstein College of Medicine and from the University of Washington suggest that HPV may eventually be cleared, or rooted out altogether, in most people with well-functioning immune systems. However, in at least some cases the virus apparently does remain in the body indefinitely, able to produce symptoms if the immune system weakens.

7. Myth: Older women don't need Pap smears.

Unfortunately, this myth is shared by many women and health care providers alike. Women who are past reproductive age may no longer visit a gynecologist, believing that they no longer need regular Paps. In many cases, no other provider recognizes the need for continued Pap screening. Data from the 1992 National Health Interview Survey indicate that one-half of all women age 60 and older have not had a Pap smear in the past three years.

The result can be deadly: One in four cases of cervical cancer, and 41% of deaths, occur in women age 65 and older. Continued Paps may be recommended because HPV can recur even after years of latency.

However, according the guidelines published by the American Cancer Society in 2002, women age 70 and older may discontinue screening if they have 3 or more normal Pap tests, and no abnormal tests in the last 10 years. What's best for you? Speak with your health care provider to see what is recommended, given your own medical history.

8. Myth: Treatment of warts means they are no longer contagious.

Unfortunately, medical opinion is not settled on this point. The closest to a consensus might be phrased as, "Don't be too sure." Transmission of HPV poses a major challenge to researchers, not only because it involves sexual behavior, which people may or may not feel free to talk about, but also because HPV's long and variable period of latency makes it virtually impossible to trace back to a specific partner.

When considering the infectiousness of treated or untreated warts, therefore, researchers must fall back on indirect observations and on reasoning from what they do know about this virus.

Some specialists think that removing genital warts may lower the risk of transmission, since it "de-bulks" the areas of tissue that contain infectious particles. But since the area surrounding any visible warts is also likely to contain infectious HPV particles, removing the warts cannot eliminate the risk.

A person may have good reasons for wanting his or her genital warts removed--they may be uncomfortable physically or psychologically. But removing warts cannot guarantee that the risk of transmission is removed.

9. Myth: A pregnant woman with genital warts is very likely to have a child with respiratory papillomatosis.

This myth refers to a possibility that, during childbirth, the baby may contract the human papillomavirus while passing through the mother's HPV-infected birth canal. The risk is real but quite small, and has been associated with only two specific types of HPV: 6 and 11. If a baby does contract HPV during birth, and if the infection persists, it may cause the child to develop lesions on the vocal cords that can interfere with breathing. This condition, known as respiratory papillomatosis, can be treated.

Delivery by cesarean section offers a baby some protection against HPV infection, but not a guarantee. Overall, the risk of respiratory papillomatosis for the baby is far smaller than the general risk of complications arising from a C-section. Pregnant women with genital warts should discuss the risks and options with their physician well before their due date and decide for themselves what they would like to do.

10. Myth: Lesbians don't need regular Pap smears.

This myth is based on an overly simple view of how HPV can be transmitted. Certainly, penile-vaginal sex can pass the virus along from one partner to another, but HPV can be passed through other forms of skin-to-skin contact as well.

The most recent evidence for this comes from a study under way at the University of Washington, which has found a number of genital HPV infections among lesbian women—even in some women who had never had sex with a man. Genital HPV in lesbians has not yet been extensively studied, but researchers suspect the prevalence rates will be lower than among heterosexuals.

Even so, the rates will not be low enough to rule out the risk of cervical cancer altogether, so a regularly scheduled Pap smear is a smart health measure for gay and straight women alike.

11. Myth: If a woman has an abnormal Pap, her male partner should get an HPV test.

Based on our experience with other infections, this would seem like a good idea. However, thus far there is no diagnostic test that can accurately determine whether a man is carrying an HPV infection. And even if he does, there is no way to treat him for the virus.

According to recent guidelines drafted by the CDC, "examination of sex partners is not necessary" as follow-up to an abnormal Pap smear. It's certainly possible--even likely--that the partner is or has been infected with the virus, although highly unlikely that he will ever show any symptoms. Nor is it possible to determine whether he can spread HPV to a future partner.

However, if a woman has external genital warts, her partner may still consider scheduling a medical exam. It may be useful for a male partner to talk with a health care provider to gain more information. And of course, if a man starts to notice symptoms of his own, such as unexplained bumps or lesions in his genital area, he should get medical attention at once.

12. Myth: If I've always used condoms, I'm not at risk for HPV.

Unfortunately, this is a dangerous myth that offers a false sense of security. Used correctly, condoms are very effective against STDs such as gonorrhea and HIV that are spread through bodily fluids. However, they are likely to be less protective against STDs that spread through skin-to-skin contact, such as HPV and herpes.

The reason is simply that condoms do not cover the entire genital area of either sex. They leave the vulva, anus, perineal area, base of the penis, and scrotum uncovered, and contact between these areas can transmit HPV. Spermicides probably do not stop HPV. In lab studies, spermicides failed to kill the human papillomavirus.

That is not to say condoms are useless. Studies have shown condom use can lower the risk of acquiring HPV infection, as well as help prevent other STDs and unintended pregnancy. For these reasons, condoms should play an important part in any new or non-monogamous sexual relationship.

HPV: Get the Facts

External Genital Warts

What are the symptoms of genital warts?

Only certain types of HPV cause genital warts. Other types, not related to genital warts, can cause abnormal cell changes on the genital skin, usually on a female's cervix.

What do warts look like?

Genital warts appear as growths or bumps. Warts may be raised or flat, single or multiple, small or large. They tend to be flesh-colored or whitish in

45

appearance. Warts usually do not cause itching, burning, or pain.

Often, genital warts are so small that they cannot be seen with the naked eye. This is sometimes called "subclinical warts." Therefore, a person may not even know he or she has the type or types of HPV that cause genital warts.

The types of HPV that cause raised external genital warts are not linked with cancer, and these types are usually harmless.

Where can genital warts appear?

Females

Vulva (entire outer female genital area)

In or around the vagina

In or around the anusGroin (where the genital area meets the inner thigh)

Cervix (less common than external warts)

Males

Penis

Scrotum (Testicular)

In or around the anus

Groin (where the genital area meets the inner thigh)

How often can episodes of genital warts occur?

•Some people only have one episode, while others have recurrences

•When warts are present, the virus is considered active

•When warts are gone, the virus is latent (sleeping) in the skin cells - it may or may not be contagious at this time

•Genital warts may or may not return after the first episode

•A healthy immune system is usually able to clear the virus, or suppress it, over time.

•Warts may appear within several weeks after sex with someone who has the wart-types of HPV, or it may take several months or years to appear. Or, warts may never appear.

This makes it hard to know exactly when or from whom someone got the virus.

How can a person get genital warts?

Any person who is sexually active can get genital warts.

The types of HPV that cause genital warts are usually spread by direct skin-to-skin contact during vaginal, anal, or possibly oral sex with someone who has this infection.

Very little is known about passing subclinical HPV to sex partners. HPV may be more likely transmitted when warts are present, but the virus can be transmitted even when there are no visible symptoms.

The types of HPV that cause genital warts are usually different from those causing warts on other body parts, such as the hands. People do not get genital warts by touching warts on their hands or feet.

Warts on other parts of the body, such as the hands, are caused by different types of HPV.

Warts are not commonly found in the mouth, so some experts believe that transmission through oral sex is not as likely as with genital-to-genital or genital-to-anal contact.

How can a person find out if they have genital warts?

Sometimes, warts can be very hard to see. Also, it can be hard to tell the difference between a wart and normal bumps on the genital area. If someone thinks he or she has warts or have been exposed to HPV, they should go to a doctor or clinic. A doctor or nurse will check more closely and may use a magnifying lens to find smaller warts.

A biopsy is not necessary for diagnosing genital warts. This is only done if the bump is unusual looking or discolored.

To look for warts or other abnormal tissue, doctors or nurses may put acetic acid (vinegar) on the genitals. This causes warts to turn white and makes them easier to see, especially if they are viewed through a magnifying lens such as a colposcope. However, the vinegar can sometimes cause other normal bumps to be highlighted, so this method of diagnosis can be misleading.

There are no blood tests clinically available to diagnose a person for HPV.

How can someone reduce the risk of getting genital warts?

Any person who is sexually active can come across this common virus. Ways to reduce the risk are:

• Not having sex with anyone.

• Having sex only with one partner who has sex only with you. People who have many sex partners are at higher risk of getting other STDs.

• If someone has visible symptoms of genital warts, he or she should not have sexual activity until the warts are removed. This may help to lower the risk of giving the virus.

•Condoms (rubbers), used the right way from start to finish each time of having sex may help provide protection - but only for the skin that is covered by the condom. Condoms do not cover all genital skin, so they don't protect 100%.

•Spermicidal foams, creams, jellies (and condoms coated with spermicide) are not proven to be effective in preventing HPV and may cause microscopic abrasions that make it easier to contract STDs. Spermicides are not recommended for routine use.

•When someone has HPV, they are not likely to be re-infected if exposed again to the same type. This is probably due to the immune system's response to the virus.

However, it is possible to be infected with a different type of HPV from a new partner.

•It is important for partners to understand the "entire picture" about HPV so that both people can make informed decisions based on facts, not fear or misconceptions.

How are genital warts treated?

•While there is no medical cure for HPV, there are several treatment options available for genital warts.

•The goal of any treatment should be to remove visible genital warts to get rid of annoying symptoms. No one treatment is best for all cases.

•Treating the warts may possibly help reduce the risk of transmission to a partner who may have never been exposed to the wart-types of HPV.

•When choosing what treatment to use, the health care provider will consider the size, location and number of warts, changes in the warts, patient preference, and cost of treatment, convenience, adverse effects, and their own experience with the treatments.

•Some treatments are done in a clinic or doctor's office; others are prescription creams that can be used at home for many weeks.

Treatments done in the doctor's office include:

•Cryotherapy (freezing off the wart with liquid nitrogen). This can be relatively inexpensive, but must be done by a trained doctor or nurse.

•Podophyllin (a chemical compound that must be applied by a doctor or nurse). This is an older treatment and is not as widely used today.

•TCA (trichloracetic acid) is another chemical applied to the surface of the wart by a doctor or a nurse.

•Cutting off warts. This has the advantage of getting rid of warts in a single office visit

•Electrocautery (burning off warts with an electrical current)

•Laser therapy (using an intense light to destroy warts).This is used for larger or extensive warts, especially those that have not responded well to other treatments.

Laser can also cost a lot of money. Most doctors do not have lasers in their office and the doctor must be well-trained with this method.

•Interferon (a substance injected in to the wart). This is rarely used anymore due to extensive side effects and high cost. Less expensive therapies work just as well with fewer side effects.

IMPORTANT: Over-the-counter wart treatments should not be used in the genital area.

What about pregnancy and genital warts?

•Most pregnant women who have had genital warts previously but no longer do would be unlikely to have any complications or problems during pregnancy or birth.

•Most children are born healthy to women with a history of genital warts.

•Because of hormone changes in the body during pregnancy, warts can grow in size and number, bleed, or, in extremely rare cases, make delivery harder.

•Very rarely, babies exposed to the wart-types of HPV during birth may develop growths in the throat.

•This so seldom happens, however, that women with genital warts do not typically need to have a cesarean-section delivery unless warts are blocking the birth canal. It is important that a pregnant woman notify her doctor or clinic if she or her partner(s) has had genital warts. This way they can determine if they need to treat the warts, or not, during the pregnancy.

What Every Woman Should Know About

Cervical Cancer and the Human

Papilloma Virus

One of the best and proven steps that you can take to prevent a cancer is to have a Pap test.

The Pap test looks for changes in the cervix that might lead to cancer.

If cancer does occur, the Pap test can find it early when it is easier to treat.

Your doctor or nurse can tell you how often you should have a Pap test.

Changes in the cervix are often caused by a virus called HPV, which is short for human papilloma virus. HPV infections can lead to cervix cancer.

This document has answers to many questions women may have about: preventing cervix cancer or finding it early the Pap test the human papilloma virus (HPV) the HPV test

The most important message for women is to have regular Pap tests to help prevent cancer of the cervix from ever occurring.

What is cervix cancer?

Cancer of the cervix is cancer that begins in the cervix, the part of the womb (or uterus) that opens to the vagina.

How common is it?

Cervix cancer is rare in this country today because most women get Pap tests that find it early or before it starts.

What is a Pap test?

The Pap test helps doctors find early changes in the cervix that might lead to cancer. It is done during a pelvic exam. Abnormal results on a Pap test are common.

Do we know what causes cervix cancer?

Cervix cancer is caused by a virus called HPV.

What is HPV?

HPV is short for human papilloma (pap-ah-LO-mah) virus. This virus can cause changes in the cervix. HPV is NOT the same as HIV.

HPV is not a new virus, but we are learning more about this virus. It is not something women should be scared about. Almost everyone has had HPV at some time in their life.

How does HPV lead to cervix cancer?

HPV is spread through sex and it can cause an infection in the cervix. The infection usually doesn't last very long because your body is able to fight the infection. If the HPV doesn't go away, the virus may cause cervix cells to change and become precancer cells.

Precancer cells are not cancer. Most cells with early precancer changes return to normal on their own. Sometimes, the precancer cells may turn into cancer if they are not found and treated. Very few HPV infections lead to cervix cancer.

Who can get cervix cancer?

Because HPV is so common, any woman who has ever had sex can get cervix cancer.

However, most women who get HPV do not get cervix cancer. Women who have their Pap tests as often as they should are least likely to get cervix cancer.

Some women have a greater chance of getting cervix cancer if they: have the HPV that can cause cervix cancer and it doesn't go away, have HIV or AIDS, smoke.

Women who don't have Pap tests done at all or who do not have them as often as they should have the greatest chance of getting cervix cancer.

If I am not having sex, do I still need to get Pap tests?

Yes. Women who were sexually active in the past can still get cervix cancer.

Who can get HPV? Any man or woman who has ever had sex can get HPV. HPV is spread by sex.

Condoms do not always protect from HPV but are very helpful in protecting from otherinfections that can be spread through sex.

Are there any symptoms of HPV?

No. Most people will never know they have HPV. But if the HPV does not go away on its own, it can cause changes in the cervix cells. These changes usually show up on your Pap test.

How is HPV treated?

There is no treatment for HPV, but most HPV infections go away without treatment. Antibiotics or other medicines do not treat HPV.

There are treatments for the cell changes in the cervix that HPV can cause. If your Pap test shows cervix changes, your doctor or nurse will discuss these treatments with you, if you need them.

Will a Pap test tell me if I have HPV?

A Pap test will usually tell you if you have any cervix cell changes that could be caused by HPV.

This is the most important information for you and your doctor to know.

No test is perfect. If a Pap test does not find cell changes that are in the cervix, then usually those changes will be found during the next Pap test. So it is important to get regular Pap tests.

Is there a test for HPV? When and how is it done?

Yes, there is a test for HPV called the HPV test. For women who are 30 years or older, the HPV test can be done at the same time as the Pap test, with a second swab.

Some women with a certain type of abnormal Pap test will get an HPV test as part of their follow up. In this case the age of the woman does not matter.

If I am over 30, do I need to be tested for HPV when I get my Pap test?

No. The choice is yours. You may want to know if you have HPV. Some women may not wish to know. You might want to take this brochure with you and ask questions at the time of your next Pap test.

If you think you might want to get an HPV test, you can get more information by calling your American Cancer Society at 1-800-ACS-2345.

No matter whether you have an HPV test or not, get your Pap test.

What can I do to prepare for my Pap test?

Try not to have your Pap test during your menstrual period.

It is best if you do not douche or have sex for 48 hours before the test.

It is best if you do not use tampons, birth control foams, jellies, or other creams or medicines in the vagina for 48 hours before the test.

Remember:

Most cervix cancers can be prevented. Finding abnormal cell changes early with a Pap test can be lifesaving. Cervix cancer is rare today in women who get their Pap tests.

See a doctor or nurse and get a Pap test. Ask your doctor or nurse how often you should have your Pap test.

HPV is a virus that can lead to cervix cancer.

Almost all women who have had sex will have HPV at some time, but very few women will get cervix cancer.

Most HPV infections go away without causing cervix changes. HPV does not have any symptoms and cannot be treated. But the cell changes that HPV can cause in the cervix can be treated.

HPV that does not go away over many years can lead to cervix cancer.

How to cure warts naturally in 5 days

My son had plantar warts for years and despite treatments from the doctor and chiropodist, nothing seemed to work. An elderly lady told us to try

CLEAR Nail varnish, well why not, he had tried everything else. Every morning and night he dabbed the varnish on and within a week they had all gone (He cleaned the old varnish off every two days BTW by peeling it off, no knives) don't ask me how it worked but it did. Hope this might help someone Regards ConnieD.

TIP: Genital warts are hard to detect at first, but a vinegar wash makes them more obvious. If you suspect that you have warts, soak a cloth with a mixture of one quarter vinegar and three quarter water and apply it to the affected area. After two minutes, genital warts usually turn white on top.

Mix Castor oil and baking soda and make a paste with the two ingredients, apply the mixture on every night and cover it with bandage, this may remove the wart in two to three weeks.

Banana peel contains a substance that is highly effective at destroying warts.

Many dermatologists recommend it. Place a small piece of banana peel against the wart and hold it in place with a bandage. Change the peel once or twice daily. Repeat for two weeks or until wart is gone.

Crush and apply a small amount of garlic directly on the wart avoiding the surrounding skin. Hold it in place with a bandage and leave it in place for 24 hours change the garlic and bandage leave it for another 24 hours. Blisters should then form, remove the bandage and wash the skin with the antiseptic skin wash. The wart should disappear within 3 to 5 days. Garlic contains protein-digesting, antiviral properties which makes it powerful and very effective to remove warts.

Topical Skin wash for warts.

2 tsp. confrey leaves.

2 tbs.. marshmallow leaves.

1 tbs.. dried yarrow.

1 cup of boiling water.

Mix herbs and cover with boiling water. Steep for 30 minutes, strain. Wash area with this solution.

After washing the skin apply Fresh Aloe Vera juice directly to the warts. Aloe Vera has both antibacterial and antiviral properties which is essential for genital warts.

Proteolytic Enzymes:

Papaya (papain), Pineapple (bromelain), banana peel and figs contain enzymes that digest and dissolve warts in a safe manner.

The fresh plant, sap (figs) or concentrate (papain) can be applied; any of these can be taped to the skin for several hours.

Milkweed a weed that is wide spread across North America; the fresh milky sap of the leaf or stem is applied directly to warts once a day. Usually works

dramatically; non-irritating, does not affect normal skin.

Increase the amount of sulfur-containing amino acids in your diet by eating more asparagus, citrus fruits, eggs, garlic, and onions.

The five day Wart removing oil treatment

½ ounce castor oil

¼ teaspoon Thuja essential oil.

¼ teaspoon tea tree essential oil.

800 International units Vitamin E oil.

Combine ingredients. The vitamin E is used to speed healing and it can be obtained by opening two 400IU capsules.

First, protect the skin around the wart with some salve, leaving the wart itself exposed. Carefully apply the mixture with a cotton swab 4 times a day. Apply it only to the wart itself this is very important because Thuja is an extremely strong formula that can burn sensitive skin.

Natural Remedies to boost the immune system

This is the most important part about fighting warts from the inside-out. The remedies you are about to learn are famous for fighting viruses like the HPV. These remedies should be used in combination with the five day wart removing oil treatment.

IMPORTANT: I do not guarantee the results of the wart removing oil treatment if you don't use the remedies to boost the immune system in combination.

First, let's learn a little bit about the immune system:

Sixty five years ago medical scientists promised us that infections caused by bacteria and others would be a thing of the past due to the new discovery of patented pharmaceutical drugs. This very brave statement was made and almost automatically more than half of the herbs recommended in the U.S. Pharmacopoeia were taken off to be replaced with these chemical drugs. I wish I could tell you that the promised was kept and that now we live in an infection free world, but this is not so. We are all familiar with the enormous amounts and resistance of bacteria. Antibiotics have not live up to their promised; to the contrary they have become a problem in itself, by over use and side effects that cause liver, kidney, nervous and immune system damage.

Modern conventional medicine battles diseases directly by means of drugs, surgery, radiation and their therapies, but true health can be attained only by maintaining a healthy properly functioning immune system.

It is the immune system that fights off disease-causing microorganisms and it engineers the healing process. The immune system is the key to fighting every kind of insult to the body, from

that little shaving scratch to the gigantic amount of viruses the constantly try to invade our bodies. Even the aging process may be related to a deteriorated immune system.

Weakening of the immune system makes us vulnerable to every type of illness that affects humans. Some common signs of impaired immune functions include fatigue, lassitude, repeated infections, inflammation, allergic reactions, slow wound healing, chronic diarrhea and infections related to overgrowth of benign organisms already present in the body, such as oral thrush, vaginal yeast infections and other fungal infections. It is calculated that a normal adult gets an average of two colds per year. People suffering from colds more than the average are likely to have some sort of immune deficiency. Dark circles could be directly related to an immune system malfunction.

Explaining what the immune system is the hard part. The immune system it is not an organ but an interaction between many organs, structures and substances with the task of recognizing or differencing from things that belong and those that don't belong to the body, and then neutralizing or destroying the ones that are foreign.

The immune system is like no other bodily system, the patrolling and protecting tasks of the immune system are share by white cells, bone marrow, the lymphatic vessels and organs, specialized cells found and various body tissues, and specialized substances, called serum factors, that are present in the blood. Ideally, all of these components work together to protects the body against diseases.

To boost and protect your immune system I recommend a list of herbs, vitamins, supplements and special recipes that have shown remarkable results throughout the years.

Astragalus boosts the immune system and generates anticancer cells in the body. It is also a powerful antioxidant and protects the liver from toxins. This makes this plant ideal for people suffering from dark circles due to liver problems and depressed immune system.

IMPORTANT: Do not take this herb if fever is present.

Baybarry has antibiotic effects for sore throat, coughs, colds and flu.

Garlic is effective against at least 30 types of bacteria, viruses, parasites and fungi. It has anti-inflammatory and astringent properties.

Echinacea boosts the immune system and enhances lymphatic function.

Goldenseal strengthens the immune system, cleanses and detoxifies the body. It has anti bacteria properties.

In a small town called Chirchik, Russia, a flu epidemic swept the town. When many adults and children did not get sick scientists wanted to know why they were immune to the disease. It turns out that all of them used the berries from an herb called Shizandra.

Immune System Booster

2 cups of water.

1 tsp. echinacea root.

½ tsp. chamomile leaves.

½ tsp. shizandra berries.

½ tsp. peppermint leaves.

Immune Tincture.

½ tsp. Echinacea root tincture.

½ tsp. pau d'arco bark tincture.

½ tsp. Siberian ginseng root tincture.

½ tsp. licorice root tincture.

½ tsp. astragalus root tincture.

½ tsp. bupleurum root tincture.

Combine all these ingredients. If you have evidence of a depressed immune system, take 3 tsp. of the formula daily for up to 5 days. Double the dose during an infection.

Include in the diet chlorella, garlic and pearl barley. These foods contain germanium, a trace element beneficial for the immune system. Also giant red kelp contains iodine, calcium, iron, carotene, protein, riboflavin and vitamin C, which are necessary for the immune system's functional integrity.

Vitamin C may be the single most important nutrient for the immune system. It is essential for the formation of adrenal hormones and the production of lymphocytes. It also has direct effect on bacteria and viruses. Vitamin C should be taken with bioflavonoids, natural plant

substances that enhance absorption and reinforce the action of this vitamin.

Shiitake (she-TAH-kee) mushrooms may be a new item in many American markets, but they have been a staple of the oriental diet for centuries. Shiitakes are the second most-consumed mushrooms in the world. Their pungent, woodsy flavor, nutritional value and health benefits attract gardeners, gourmets, and mushroom lovers, even at $12-26 a pound.

Shiitakes ("shii" is Japanese for oak and "take" means mushroom) are delicious, with a meaty texture and four times the flavor of white button mushrooms. Shiitakes provide high levels of protein (18% by mass), potassium, niacin and B vitamins, calcium, magnesium and phosphorus. The mushroom has all essential amino acids.

Shiitakes have natural antiviral and immunity-boosting properties and are used nutritionally to fight viruses, lower cholesterol and regulate blood pressure. Researchers S. Suzuki and Oshima found that a raw shiitake eaten daily for one week lowered serum cholesterol by 12%. Concentrated forms of lentinan, a shiitake extract, have been used to treat cancer, AIDS, diabetes, fibrosystic breast disease and other conditions with impressive results.

Take 300 to 500 milligrams twice a day to keep wart from coming back.

MOST POPULAR HOME REMEDIES WARTS

Home Remedies warts #1: Fresh Aloe vera juice is applied directly to dissolve warts and tone the skin.

Home Remedies warts #2: Proteolytic Enzymes:

Papaya (papain), Pineapple (bromelain), banana peel and figs contain enzymes that digest and dissolve warts in a safe manner.

Home Remedies warts #3: The fresh plant, sap (figs) or concentrate (papain) can be applied; any of these can be taped to the skin for several hours.

Home Remedies warts #4: Milkweed a weed that is wide spread across North America; the fresh milky sap of the leaf or stem is applied directly to warts once a day.

Home Remedies warts #5: Increase the amount of sulfur-containing amino acids in your diet by eating more asparagus, citrus fruits, eggs, garlic, and onions.

HOME REMEDIES WARTS

One of the most skin conditions are common warts these unsightly bumps that usually appear in hands, face, neck and décolleté.

They are not painful, even if they are too large can become annoying, but are associated with ugliness. They are common in children and adolescents and usually fade over time. Conventional wisdom has a host of remedies against them.

HOME REMEDIES WARTS TREATMENT

1 MILK FRESH FIG

A simple way to remove warts short term is the implementation of milk fresh fig. We need fresh fig 1 for each wart.

Preparation

Pumping of fresh fig.

How to apply

Apply milk of fig on each wart, but within its outline.

Cover the area with a bandage or gauze.

Keep the poultice for 8 hours.

Repeat the cure for 9 days, renewing the milk daily.

ELIMINATE WARTS NATURALLY

They are presented in various sizes and shapes and are usually located on the hands and fingers, but sometimes may occur elsewhere in the body.

This is because it is spread by direct contact. That is, for the contact of a body part with another. Touching a wart on your hand, you can take the virus with the fingers and transfer it to another part of the skin surface

Those who appear in the feet are called plantar warts are very painful and making the person unable to walk properly. It must be very careful with genital warts which require medical attention.

Warts Remedies

Home Remedies warts # 1: Rub the wart with a piece of garlic or garlic juice.

Home Remedies warts # 2: Immerse plantar warts in hot water every night.

Home Remedies warts # 3: Apply vitamin E oil, essential oil of cloves or sage, aloe vera (aloe) directly on the wart.

Home Remedies warts # 4: Soak several slices of lemon in apple cider with a little salt and marinate for two weeks. After that time, take the slices of lemon and rub over the wart.

Home Remedies warts # 5: Rub a piece of chalk, a raw potato or banana peel on the wart.

Home Remedies warts # 6: Apply a drop of castor oil to the wart twice daily and cover with a bandage or tape.

Home Remedies warts # 7: Form a thick paste with a spoonful of castor oil with baking soda. Apply the paste a couple of times a day and then cover with a bandage.

Powerful Homeopathic Remedies (Optional)

If you are the kind of individual that prefers homeopathic medicine, you can use the treatment below to resolve warts:

Days 1 – 4: Take one dose of Thuja 30x or 9c twice a day.

Days 4 – 9: Take one dose of Nitricum acidum 12x or 6c twice a day.

If the wart has not cleared after nine days, consider one of the symptoms-specific remedies that follow.

If the wart is dry and itchy, take one dose of Antimonium crudum 12x or 6c three time daily for three days.

Use Causticum for warts that bleed easily, are flat and are mostly found on the fingers.

Take one dose of Causticum 12x or 5c three times daily for up to three days.

Mercurius cyanatus is especially helpful for plantar warts. Take one dose of mercurius cyanatus 12x or 5c twice a day for up to five days.

Apply homeopathic Thuja ointment to the warts once a day for three weeks.

At-home prescription creams:

•Podofilox cream or gel (Condylox®). This is a self-applied treatment for external genital warts. It may be less expensive than treatment done in a health care provider's office, is easy to use and is safe, but it must be used for about 4 weeks.

•Imiquimod cream (Aldara®). This is also a self-applied treatment for external genital warts. It is safe, effective and easy to use. This cream is different than other commonly-used treatments, which work by destroying the wart tissue.

Aldara actually boosts the immune system to fight HPV.